Medicare Made Easy

William Wells

A wise man takes the shortest route to his destination.

----Will Naylor, 1953

Table of Contents

Prologue i
Medicare Made Easy 3
How to sign up for Part A and Part B 5
Part D – Prescription Drugs 7
What is ObamaCare? 7
2014 Medicare Part D Benefit Parameters 11
Medigap/Medicare Supplement Plan 14
Medicare Supplement Plan F covers 15
Reasons to have a Medigap/Medicare Supplement Plan 16
Part D – Prescription Drugs 16
Medicare Election Periods 18
Annual (OPEN) Election Period 19
Special Election Periods 21
Scope of Sales Appointment Confirmation Form 23
Diagnostic Services 25
PACE, PACENET, and PACE Plus Medicare 28
The Affordable Care Act 29
Veterans' Benefits 30
Creating an Online Account with Social Security 30
Selecting a Drug Plan 31
Prescription Drug Plan Formularies 33
What is Step Therapy? 34
Why is Medicare so confusing? 36

Prologue

Medicare Made Easy describes the nuts and bolts of Medicare and Health Insurance in an easily understandable, orderly and readable fashion. This edition is a primer for Medicare and Health Insurance for 2013 and 2014. Things you need to know about Medicare and Health Insurance are covered. Every day, all across America, approximately ten thousand people will turn sixty-five years of age and become eligible for Medicare. It will continue at this rate until the year 2022.

The author wrote this book because when he turned sixty-five years of age he was totally confused and perplexed by all the different health insurance programs and terminologies. He did not even know the difference between Medigap Plans/Medicare Supplement Plans and Medicare Advantage Plans. He figured that there had to be some easy way to explain Medicare and Health Insurance Plans so they were easily understandable.

Medicare Made Easy

Medicare is Health Insurance for persons sixty-five and older, or persons who are deemed disabled by social security for twenty-five months.

An individual is eligible for Medicare benefits at age sixty-five, if they have worked and paid into payroll taxes for at least forty quarters, or ten years, or those who may draw these benefits from a spouse. Three months before you turn sixty-five, the month you turn sixty-five, and three months after you turn sixty-five you are eligible to sign up for Medicare. There is a seven month window to sign up for Medicare.

If you are deemed disabled by Social Security, there is a waiting period of twenty-four months prior to receiving your Medicare benefits.

The Centers for Medicare and Medicaid Services (CMS) governs the actions of Medicare, Medicaid, Medicare Advantage, Part D Prescription Drug Program, and Children's Health Insurance Program.

CMS approves most marketing and informational materials about Medicare that the public receives. The main focus is to protect those who are eligible for Medicare.

The function of CMS is to protect Medicare beneficiaries as well as provide information and guidelines. CMS sets standards and policies for companies involved with Medicare.

The four parts of Medicare are described below:

Part A – Hospital Coverage – also covers Skilled Nursing Facility, Home Health Care and Hospice.

Part B – Medical Coverage – Has a premium and deductible. The premium for 2013 is $104.90 per month for 2013 and will remain the same for 2014, and the deductible for 2013 is $147 and is the same for 2014. Part B covers Doctor's Services, Medical Services, Supplies, Diagnostic Tests, Outpatient Therapy, Outpatient Mental Health, Some Preventive Services, Emergency Services, and Ambulance Services. After the deductible amount is met, then Medicare will pay 80% of APPROVED charges, and you will owe the remaining 20%.

Creditable Coverage and Late Enrollment Penalty - There is a 10% per year penalty assessed to any Medicare beneficiary who declines to have Part B and does not have creditable coverage. Creditable coverage would be considered coverage through an employer or the employer of a spouse.

How to sign up for Part A and Part B

Apply online at **www.ssa.gov** or visit your local Social Security office or call Social Security at **1-800-772-1213**.

Medicare Part C

Medicare Part C Plans are known as Medicare Advantage Plans. These are private plans run through Medicare that, by law, must be equivalent to regular **Part A** coverage and **Part B** coverage. There are lots of variations among **Part C** plans.

Part D – Drug Coverage

If you have any questions about your coverage, talk to your doctor, pharmacist or other health care provider about Medicare coverage for services and supplies to see if Medicare covers them. When you go for an appointment, have your Medicare Card and your insurance cards with you. When you register for an appointment with a doctor's office or other medical facility and they ask for your Medicare Card and insurance card, usually they advise you what is covered under your plans and what out of pocket expenses you might except if any. Documents they have you sign should spell all this out.

Part C - Medicare Advantage Plans operate under Medicare and take the place of Original Medicare. Many plans offer additional diversified coverage for less money like prescription coverage, eye care, and gym plans to name a few of the additional things offered. At any time an individual can opt out of a Medicare Advantage Plan and return to Original Medicare. Eighty-seven cents of every dollar paid to Medicare Advantage insurance premiums goes to care and benefits.

Medicare Advantage Plans are provided by private companies contracted with Centers for Medicare and Medicaid Services (CMS). They cover all of Parts A, B and in most cases D, and typically include more benefits than Original Medicare. You will never lose your Original Medicare by joining a Medicare Advantage Plan. These plans are options for addressing health care needs that may not be paid by Original Medicare Parts A and B or Medicare Supplements and are offered by private companies contracted by Medicare to provide coverage.

Medigap/Medicare Supplement Plan – A supplement plan is an insurance policy purchased from a private company which may cover some or all the Medicare deductibles and 20% coinsurance. The benefits of these policies are mandated by federal law to be standardized, but the premium amount may vary. Premiums must be paid regardless of utilization of benefits and services. Medigap is another name for a Medicare Supplement Plan.

Part D – Prescription Drugs - Five out of six people sixty-five and older are taking at least one medication with most older adults taking three or more. Not all drugs are covered by Medicare Part D. The list of covered drugs is in a companies' formulary.

Part D became part of the Medicare program in January 2006 through legislation passed by Congress in 2003. This was the first time in the history of Medicare that prescriptions had been covered. You must buy your Part D from a private company and copays, coinsurance, premiums and formularies will vary from company to company. A Formulary must include at least two drugs in categories and classes of most commonly prescribed drugs to people with Medicare.

To participate in a Medigap/Medicare Supplement Plan or a Medicare Advantage plan, you must have Medicare Part B.

What is ObamaCare?

The 2010 Affordable Care Act (ACA) is Obama Care. The healthcare exchanges are a pillar of the act. They will allow uninsured people to buy highly regulated subsidized insurance plans on new statewide websites. About twenty-four million people are expected to enroll in the exchanges by 2013. Millions of people will qualify for subsidies under the law.

Obama Care is the unofficial name for the Patient Protection and Affordable Care Act which was signed into law on March 23, 2010. In a more general sense Obama Care and The Health Care for America Plan or any such name is a reference to the Affordable Care Act.

Although the Affordable Care Act (Obama Care) was signed into law in 2010, the health care reforms it enacts roll out year- by- year until 2022. Many of the biggest reforms don't kick in until 2014.

ObamaCare is designed to ensure that health care coverage is available to any legal U.S. resident who cannot otherwise obtain quality healthcare through their employer. Your access to health care is no longer in the hands of health insurance companies. If you are on Medicare, you are not eligible for ObamaCare. The Affordable Care Act is primarily for people aged twenty to sixty-four. Go to the following website for more detailed information: **http://obamacarefacts.com/whatis-obamacare.php**

To sign up for ObamaCare, go to: **Healthcare.gov**

Using the marketplace at Healthcare.gov will help you complete the entire application process from beginning to end with information you provide over the phone, including reviewing your options and helping you enroll in a plan. It will also answer questions as you fill out an online or paper application. The service is available 24/7. **The Health Insurance Marketplace** contact number is: **1-800-318-2596, TTY: 1-855-889-4325.**

To check healthcare plans and prices, go to **HealthCare. premium-estimates** gov/find-. These costs will not reflect the discount you get based on household size and income.

Also, you can apply in person by working with a counselor in your area. Go to **LocalHelp.Healthcare.gov** and put in your Zip Code. If your state has its own exchange, you will be directed to that website.

You can apply by mail by printing out an application from the website **Healthcare.gov** and mail it in.

A word of caution – make sure that the website you are dealing with is a legitimate website. If in doubt, call 1-800-318-2596 to verify that the site you are using is not a fraudulent website.

You must provide an accurate estimate for 2014 income. Most people will be getting a tax credit to help pay their premiums. The credits are based on your income and keyed to the premium for a bench mark plan known as the **second-lowest Silver plan** in your area.

You will have four levels of insurance to consider: bronze, silver, gold and platinum. Plans at every level cover the same benefits and have a cap of $6,350 a year in out-of-pocket expenses for an individual, $12,700 for families.

Bronze plans have the lowest premiums but cover only sixty per cent of medical costs on average. Policyholders will pay the difference, up to the annual out-of-pocket cap.

Platinum plans have the highest premiums, and they cover ninety per cent of costs. Young adults to age 30 can pick a low cost catastrophic plan, but a tax credit does not apply to this plan. You must have health insurance by March 17, 2014 or you will have to pay a penalty to the IRS.

Make sure your doctors and hospitals are in the plan you choose. Your share of the premium could be lower and even cost nothing because the credit is keyed to the cost of the sliver plan, which is usually more expensive.

In addition to your tax credit, see if you are eligible for cost-sharing subsidies. Extra help is available for low incomes, but only with a silver plan.

AGE 26 – The plan allows young people to stay on their parents' insurance plans until age 26. It also covers dependents, step-children, adopted children and some foster children.

Many seniors think they will be able to enroll in a health or prescription drug plan through a public health insurance exchange which is not the case. A public health insurance exchange is only for uninsured people under the age of 65.

2014 Medicare Part D Benefit Parameters

The **Centers for Medicare & Medicaid Services** has released the Medicare Part D standard benefit parameters and the cost thresholds and limits for qualified retiree prescription drug plans for 2014. The standard benefit parameters will drop from 2013 by approximately 4%. The IRS has also provided important guidance on the change in taxation of retiree drug subsidies that is effective in 2013. Plan sponsors that want to remain qualified for the employer retiree drug subsidy will have to determine if their 2014 prescription drug coverage is at least actuarially equivalent to the standard Medicare Part D coverage.

	2013	2014
Deductible	$ 325.00	$ 310.00
Initial coverage limit	$ 2,970.00	$ 2,850.0
Out-of-pocket (OOP) threshold	$ 4,750.00	$ 4,550.0
Minimum copay (catastrophic portion of benefit)	$ 2.65	$ 2.55
	$ 6.60	$ 6.35
Generic/preferred drug		
All other drugs		

In 2014 Part D, in the Deductible Period you pay 100% of prescriptions up to $310. In the Initial Phase from $310 to $2850, you pay copays and coinsurance. In the donut hole, the out-of-pocket threshold, you will pay a reduced rate from $2,850 to $4,550. The catastrophic level is above $4,550 where you will pay $2.55 for generic or preferred drugs. All other drugs will cost $6.35 per prescription.

Many seniors think they will be able to enroll in a health or prescription drug plan through a public health insurance exchange which is not the case. A public health insurance exchange is only for uninsured people under the age of 65.

Part C - Medicare Advantage Plans operate under Medicare and take the place of Original Medicare. Many plans offer additional diversified coverage for less money like prescription coverage, eye care, and gym plans to name a few of the additional things offered. At any time an individual can opt out of a Medicare Advantage Plan and return to Original Medicare. Eighty-seven cents of every dollar paid to Medicare Advantage insurance premiums goes to care and benefits.

Medicare Advantage Plans are provided by private companies contracted with Centers for Medicare and Medicaid Services. They cover all of Parts A, B and in most cases D. They typically include more benefits than Original Medicare. You will never lose your Original Medicare by joining a Medicare Advantage Plan. These plans are options for addressing health care needs that may not be paid by Original Medicare Parts A and B or Medicare Supplements and are offered by private companies contracted by Medicare to provide coverage.

Medigap/Medicare Supplement Plan – A supplement plan is an insurance policy purchased from a private company which may cover some or all the Medicare deductibles and 20% coinsurance. The benefits of these policies are mandated by federal law to be standardized, but the premium amount may vary. Premiums must be paid regardless of utilization of benefits and services. Medigap is another name for a Medicare Supplement Plan.

Medicare Supplement Plan F is the most comprehensive plan and the most widely selected Medigap/Medicare Supplement Plan.

With Medicare Supplement Plan F, you get the most complete Medigap coverage available. It is the only Medicare Supplement insurance plan that covers both **Part B Medicare deductible and Medicare Excess Charges**. An excess charge is the difference between what a doctor or provider charges and the amount Medicare will pay. Because the plan covers costs in excess of Medicare-approved amounts, you will likely have no-out- of – pocket costs for hospital and doctor's office care with this plan. Plus, most importantly, you get to choose your own doctors.

Medicare Supplement Plan F covers:

1) Hospitalization: pays Part A coinsurance plus coverage for 365 additional days after Medicare benefits stop.
2) Medical Expenses: pays Part B coinsurance – generally 20 percent of Medicare- approved expenses – or copayments for hospital outpatient services.
3) Blood: pays for the first three pints of blood each year.
4) Skilled nursing facility care.
5) Medicare Part A deductible for hospitalization.
6) Medicare Part B deductible for medical and hospital outpatient expenses.
7) Medicare Part B Excess Charges – This is the difference between what a doctor or provider charges and the amount Medicare will pay up to Medicare's limiting amount
8) Travel-abroad medical emergency help

Why is it important to buy a **Medicare Supplement Policy/Medigap Policy** when you are first eligible?

Applying for Medigap during your open enrollment period, you can buy any Medigap policy the company sells, even if you have health problems for the same price as people with good health.

Applying after your open enrollment period, there is no guarantee that an insurance company will sell you a Medigap policy if you don't meet the medical underwriting requirements. As long as you pay your premium, you can never be cancelled.

Reasons to have a Medigap/Medicare Supplement Plan

1. Allows you to choose a doctor of your choice

2. Covers skilled nursing facilities expenses not covered by Medicare

3. Covers hospital expenses not covered by Medicare

4. Covers durable medical equipment like a motorized wheel chair

5. Covers foreign travel for emergency care

For information about Medicare health care insurance, contact:

MedicareMadeEasy7@gmail.com or 610-287-7232.

Part D – Prescription Drugs - Five out of six people sixty-five and older are taking at least one medication with most taking three or more. Not all drugs are covered by Medicare Part D. The list of covered drugs is in a companies' formulary.

Part D became part of the Medicare program in January 2006 through legislation passed by Congress in 2003. This was the first time in the history of Medicare that prescriptions had been covered. You must buy your Part D from a private company **and copays, and coinsurance and premiums and formularies will vary from company to company.**

A formulary must include at least two drugs in categories and classes of most commonly prescribed drugs for people with Medicare.

Compare Medicare Part D Plans - Don't choose a plan based on premium alone. First check the Medicare Part D formulary - **Basic, Most Common Drugs, and Enhanced**.

If all your drugs are not on the formulary, it is not a good plan for you. Drugs are not placed in the same tier by different companies.

Compare copayments and coinsurance amounts between plans. Also, what kind of deductible does the plan have?

Compare mail order benefits. Premiums may not be what are published on the Medicare website – Medicare.gov.

Part D premiums are now tied to your annual income. At the poverty line, you may pay nothing. Above $85,000 and $170,000 expect to pay more.

Medicare Election Periods

1. **Initial Election Period** - This is when the beneficiary has just become eligible for Medicare or when the beneficiary becomes sixty-five years of age.

2. **Annual Election Period** - Beneficiaries can be enrolled between October 15 and December 7.

3. **Medicare Disenrollment Period** – Beneficiaries can leave their current plan between January 1 and February 14 and switch back to Original Medicare.

4. **Special Election Period(SEP)** – Beneficiaries can switch plans who qualify for enrollment under certain circumstances such as moving, dual eligibility, extra help with prescription drug costs and receiving care in an institutional setting.

Initial Election Period (ICEP)

A Medicare Beneficiary can enroll into a Medicare Advantage Plan or a Prescription Drug Plan when he or she becomes eligible for Medicare.

Eligibility can be due to any of the following:

1. Beneficiary is turning sixty-five years of age.

2. Beneficiary has a disability.

3. Beneficiary with disability is turning sixty-five years of age.
4. Beneficiary has just enrolled in Medicare Part B

Beneficiaries on disability can sign up for a Medicare Advantage Plan or a Prescription Drug Plan three months before their twenty-fifth month of disability, or in the three months after their twenty-fifth month of disability.

Annual (OPEN) Election Period

This is the biggest election period of the year. Medicare beneficiaries can join or make changes to their **Medicare Advantage or**

Prescription Drug Plans between October 15 and December 7. A beneficiary can do any of the following:

1. Change from Original Medicare to a Medicare Advantage Plan.

2. Switch from a current Medicare Advantage Plan to another Medicare Advantage Plan.

3. Switch from a Medicare Advantage Plan that doesn't offer drug coverage to a plan that does offer drug coverage or vice versa.

4. Join a Medicare Prescription Drug Plan.

5. Switch from one Medicare Prescription Drug Plan to another Medicare Prescription Drug Plan.

Medicare Advantage Disenrollment Period

Beneficiaries can leave their current plan and switch to Original Medicare between January 1 and February 14. Beneficiaries who switch to Original Medicare can join a Prescription Drug Plan to add a Part D Plan.

1. A beneficiary cannot switch from **Original Medicare** to an **Advantage Drug Plan.**

2. A beneficiary cannot switch from one **Medicare Advantage Plan** to another.

3. A beneficiary cannot switch from one **Medicare Prescription Drug Plan** to another.

4. A beneficiary cannot join, switch or drop a **Medicare Medical Savings Plan.**

Special Election Periods

When certain events happen in a beneficiary's life such as moving or losing coverage, the beneficiary can take advantage of a special election period to switch or enroll in a new plan such as the following:

1. Beneficiary moves out of his service area.

2. Beneficiary loses current coverage.

3. Beneficiary has chance to get other coverage.

4. Beneficiary's plan changes its contract with Medicare.

5. Other special circumstances.

6. When a beneficiary leaves a Medicare Cost Plan with a drug plan, a beneficiary has two months to enroll in a Part D Plan.

7. A beneficiary moving back to the United State from overseas has two months to enroll into a Medicare Advantage Plan or a Part D Plan.

8. A beneficiary released from jail has two months to sign up for a Medicare Advantage Plan or a Part D Plan.

9. A beneficiary that has dual eligibility(Medicare and Medicaid) may switch plans at any time.

10. Once a year, State Pharmaceutical Assistance Program beneficiaries can switch to a Medicare Advantage or Part D Plan.

11. Beneficiaries who no longer qualify for a Special Needs Plan (SNP) can join a Medicare Advantage Plan or Part D Plan within the three month SNP grace period.

12. A beneficiary with a severe health condition can enroll in a Chronic Special Needs Plan. Once enrolled, this eliminates the ability to make Special Election Period changes.

Scope of Sales Appointment Confirmation Form

The **Centers for Medicare and Medicaid Services** requires agents to document the scope of a marketing appointment prior to any face-to-face sales meeting to ensure understanding of what will be discussed between the agent and Medicare beneficiary or their authorized representative. All this information provided on this form is confidential and should be completed by each person with Medicare or their authorized representative.

Besides **Medigap/Medicare Supplement Plans**, the agent can discuss the following plans:

1. **Medicare Prescription Drug Plan (PDP)** – A stand-alone drug plan that adds prescription drug coverage to Original Medicare.

2. **Medicare Health Maintenance Organization(HMO)** – A Medicare Advantage Plan that provides all Original Medicare Part A and Part B health coverage and sometimes covers Part D prescription drug coverage. In most HMOs, you can only get your care from doctors or hospitals in the plan's network except in emergencies.

3. **Medicare Preferred Provider Organization (PPO) Plan** – A Medicare Advantage Plan that provides all Original Medicare Part A and Part B health coverage and sometimes covers Part D prescription drug

coverage. PPOs have network doctors and hospitals but you can also use out-of-network providers, usually at a higher cost.

4. **Medicare Fee-For-Service (PFFS) Plan** – A Medicare Advantage Plan in which you may go to any Medicare-approved doctor, hospital and provider that accepts the plan's payment, terms and conditions and agrees to treat you – not all providers will. If you join a PFFS Plan that has a network, you can see any of the network providers who have agreed to always treat plan members. You will usually pay more to see out-of-network providers.

5. **Medicare Special Needs Plan (SNP)** – A Medicare Advantage Plan that has a benefit package designed for people with special health care needs. Examples of the specific groups served include people who have both Medicare and Medicaid, people who reside in nursing homes, and people who have certain chronic medical conditions.

6. **Medicare Medical Savings Account (MSA)Plan** – MSA Plans combine a high deductible health plan with a bank account. The plan deposits money from Medicare into the account. You can use it to pay your medical expenses until your deductible is met.

7. **Medicare Cost Plan** – In a Medicare Cost Plan, you can go to providers both in and out of network. If you get services outside of the plan's network, your Medicare covered services will be paid for under Original Medicare. You will be responsible for Medicare coinsurance and deductibles:

Diagnostic Services

If you need any diagnostic services like blood tests, make sure that you schedule an appointment. A lot of appointments can be scheduled on line. If you walk-in, you could be waiting a long time before you are seen if you don't have an appointment. If you are waiting without an appointment, people with appointments go ahead of you. I know because I have waited over an hour on two occasions. The second time I walked out.

Low Income Subsidy is also known as Extra Help

A lot of people are not aware of **Extra Help** in spite of Medicare's efforts to make them aware of its benefits. A beneficiary must be entitled to Medicare Part A and/or enrolled in Medicare Part B. Beneficiary must live in one of the fifty states or the District of Columbia. The following guidelines apply for 2013 and may still apply for 2014: The beneficiary is single and has income less than $17,235 and resources less than $13,300; or beneficiary is married with no dependents and is making less than $3,265 and less than $26,380 in resources.

A checking or a savings account, stocks, bonds, mutual funds, and Individual Retirement Accounts are resources. Not counted as resources is your home, car, household items, burial plot, up to $1500 burial expenses per person, or life insurance policies.

An application for **Extra Help** does not enroll you in a Medicare prescription drug plan. You will have to enroll directly with an approved Medicare prescription drug provider for coverage. If you need information about Medicare Prescription Drug plans or how to enroll in a plan, call **1-800-633-4227 (TTY 1-877-486-2048)** or visit www.medicare.gov. In Pennsylvania, for information, you may dial **1-610-287-7232** for help with your Medicare Health Insurance needs.

To apply online for Extra Help go to: **https://secure.ssa.gov/i1020/start**.

List of documents needed for Extra Help Application:

1. Social Security Card.

2. Checking, Savings, Certificate of Deposit bank statements.

3. Investment Information: Individual Retirement Accounts, stocks, bonds, savings bonds, mutual fund, other investment statements.

4. Tax Returns.

5. Payroll Slips.

6. Most recent Social Security benefits award letters.

7. Railroad Retirement Benefits.

8. Veterans' Benefits.

9. Pensions.

Extra Help Automatic Qualification

Certain beneficiaries automatically qualify for Extra Help and they need not apply. Such beneficiaries would have Medicare and meet the following conditions:

1. Have full Medicaid coverage.

2. Receive help from their state Medicaid program paying their Part B premiums (in a Medicare Savings program).

3. Receive Supplemental Security Income (SSI) benefits.

PACE, PACENET, and PACE Plus Medicare

PACE, PACENET and PACE plus Medicare are Pennsylvania's prescription assistance programs for older adults, offering low-cost prescription medication to qualified residents, age 65 and older.

Who is Eligible?

To be eligible for PACE and PACENET: You must be 65 years of age or older. A Pennsylvania resident for at least 90 days prior to the date of application cannot be enrolled in the Department of Public Welfare's Medicaid prescription drug benefit program. PACE and PACENET eligibility is determined by your previous calendar year's income.

PACE

For a single person, total income must be $14,500 or less. For a married couple, combined total income must be $17,700 or less.

PACENET

For a single person, total income can be between $14,500 and $23,500. For a married couple, combined total income can be between $17,700 and $31,500.

PACE Plus Medicare

Under PACE Plus Medicare, PACE/PACENET coverage is supplemented by federal Medicare Part D prescription coverage and offers older Pennsylvanians the best benefits of both programs. Older adults continue to receive the same prescription benefits while, in many cases, saving more money.

The Affordable Care Act

Effective December 15, 2013, you need to have qualifying insurance or an exemption. Most people will pay a penalty to the government if they do not have a health plan. The charges are:

2014   Penalty - $95 or 1% of your taxable income.

2015   Penalty - $325 or 2% of your taxable income.

2016   Penalty - $695 or 2.5% of your taxable income.

If you choose to pay a penalty, you will not receive health insurance coverage. You will still be responsible for 100% of the cost of your own medical care. After the open enrollment period ends on March 31, 2014, you won't be able to get health insurance coverage through the Marketplace until the next annual enrollment period unless you have a qualifying life event.

Veterans' Benefits

War-time veterans who served at least ninety days of active military service may qualify for Veterans' benefits. It helps pay for long-term care, prescriptions, and other healthcare for veterans and their spouses. To find local help to apply, go to VA.gov.

Creating an Online Account with Social Security

You can create an online account with Social Security to monitor your activity. You have the ability to log in any time to access your account **www.socialsecurity.gov/myaccount** with your user name and password to access Social Security's online services. It will show you your entire history of Social Security earnings year-by-year and other important information.

APPRISE

APPRISE is Pennsylvania's State Health Insurance Assistance Program. The Pennsylvania Department of Aging created APPRISE to help Pennsylvania residents understand their Medicare and other health insurance benefits, and assist citizens in making informed decisions about their health care options. Apprise counselors can help you understand your Medicare plan choices and can help you understand different Medicare plans and answers questions about switching plans. Apprise's phone number is **1-800-783-7067**, and their website is: **www.aging.state.pa.us**.

Selecting a Drug Plan

Most drugs are not covered under Original Medicare. You can add **prescription drug coverage** to original Medicare by joining a Medicare Prescription Drug plan, or you can get all your Medicare coverage, including prescription drug coverage, by joining a Medicare Advantage Plan or a Medicare Cost Plan that offers prescription drug coverage. It is important to select the right plan.

If you have Original Medicare and a Medigap plan, you may add a stand-alone Medicare Part D Drug Plan. You cannot have a Medigap plan and a Medicare Advantage Plan at the same time. It is one or the other.

A **formulary** is a list of covered drugs in a drug plan, different companies have different formularies. In a **Medicare Advantage Plan** check out the drugs you are taking with the **Formulary** to see if the drugs you are taking are in the plan.

Formularies vary from plan-to-plan. Some plans may not include all your prescribed drugs. Some medications are not covered by any drug formulary in which case you will have to pay out- of -pocket or seek assistance to pay for those drugs.

It is important to enroll in a drug plan when you become eligible so that you are not penalized. After you have found a plan suitable for you, compare it to the Retail Pharmacy Network and the Mail Order Plan. This can save you a lot of money. **Medicare.gov** rates various plans by people's experiences with them.

Find a plan that covers all your medications with the lowest costs, and you have found the plan for you.

Through this website: **www.medicare.gov**, you can learn about **Prescription Drug Plans(PDP's).**

Prescription Drug Plan Formularies

A **formulary**, or drug list, is a list of prescriptions and medications that are covered under a health care plan that provide prescription drug coverage.

Coverage Limitations

To be covered, drugs must be prescribed for a use that is approved by the **FDA** or documented in at least one of the specific peer-review compendia identified by the Centers for Medicare and Medicaid Services (CMS). You can find out if any additional prescription drug coverage limitations apply to your drugs by looking at the **Prior Authorization**. **Prior authorization** requires you or your doctor to get approval from the plan before your drug is covered.

2014 Prior Authorization Criteria

The plan requires you or your doctor to get **prior authorization** for certain drugs. This means the plan needs more information from your doctor to make sure the drug is being used correctly for a medical condition covered by Medicare. If you don't get approval, the plan may not cover the drug.

What is Step Therapy?

There are effective, lower-cost drugs that treat the same medical conditions as the drug that you may be using. You may be required to try one or more of these other drugs before the plan will cover your drug. Having tried other drugs or your doctor thinks they are not right for you, you and your doctor can ask the plan to cover this drug.

Formulary Change Notifications

Notice of Formulary Changes will be posted sixty days prior to the removal or change in the preferred or tiered cost-sharing status of a Medicare Part D drug. The posting will include:

1. Name of the affected covered Medicare Part D drug.

2. Information on whether the covered Medicare Part D drug is being removed from the formulary, or changing its preferred or tiered cost-sharing status.

3. The reason the covered Medicare Part D drug is being removed from the formulary, or changing its preferred or tiered cost-sharing status.

4. Alternative drugs in the same therapeutic category, class or cost-sharing tier, and the expected cost sharing for that drug.

5. The means by which members may obtain an updated coverage determination or an exception to a coverage determination.

Tier 1 drugs are generic. They have exactly the same active ingredients as their brand name counterparts. Your costs will be lowest with Tier 1 drugs. In Massachusetts, you are automatically given Tier 1/generic drugs unless your provider makes a special request.

Tier 2 drugs are brand name medications that are on a list of preferred drugs — also referred to as the **Preferred Formulary List (PDF)** — approved by a panel of doctors and pharmacists as safe, effective, and less expensive than other alternatives. You will pay more for Tier 2 drugs than Tier 1 drugs.

Tier 3 drugs are brand-name medications that have not been identified as an effective, lower cost medication on the formulary list. Your costs will be highest with Tier 3 drugs, and they are referred to as

non- preferred - Most people only use Tier 3 drugs when they have not gotten any results with Tier 1 or Tier 2.

Tier 4 drugs are non-preferred brand name drugs and preferred specialty drugs.

Tier 5 drugs are specialty drugs that require special dosing or administration.

Why is Medicare so confusing?

Most people need to have Medicare unless they have their own insurance plan. There is no Medicare office. Medicare is managed by the **Centers for Medicare & Medicaid Services (CMS).** Social Security works with CMS by enrolling people in Medicare. You can go to your local Social Security office to sign up. You are automatically enrolled in Medicare Plan A if you have worked forty quarters (ten years) and paid into Social Security.

Then, there are supplemental plans, Medigap, Part D – Prescription Drug Plans, Medicare Advantage plans, Supplemental Medicare plans – Plan A, Plan F, and so on. What are the costs? Is your head spinning yet?

How many advertisements did you receive from healthcare companies or their intermediaries? Did you get a Medicare booklet "Medicare and You" from the Government?

All these mailers you received about Medicare and Medicare Health Providers, did you really understand them? When I turned sixty-five, I didn't. All the Medigap A's and D's and F's totally confused me. As for the Medicare Advantage Plans, that was really confusing. Then, the Part D about prescription drug costs totally flummoxed me. I telephoned several of the major health care insurance companies, and I still could not figure it out. Finally, a nice lady with one of the major health insurance companies came to our house. She sat down and clearly and concisely explained everything to my wife and me and that was that. The rates were competitive or better than others. We signed on the dotted line.
What do you need to know to make a decision about **Medicare Coverage**? You need to know what coverage you need and what it is going to cost. It is that simple. For information about Medicare health care insurance contact: **MedicareMadeEasy7@gmail.com or 610-287-7232.**

www.ingramcontent.com/pod-product-compliance
Lightning Source LLC
Chambersburg PA
CBHW070719180526
45167CB00004B/1537